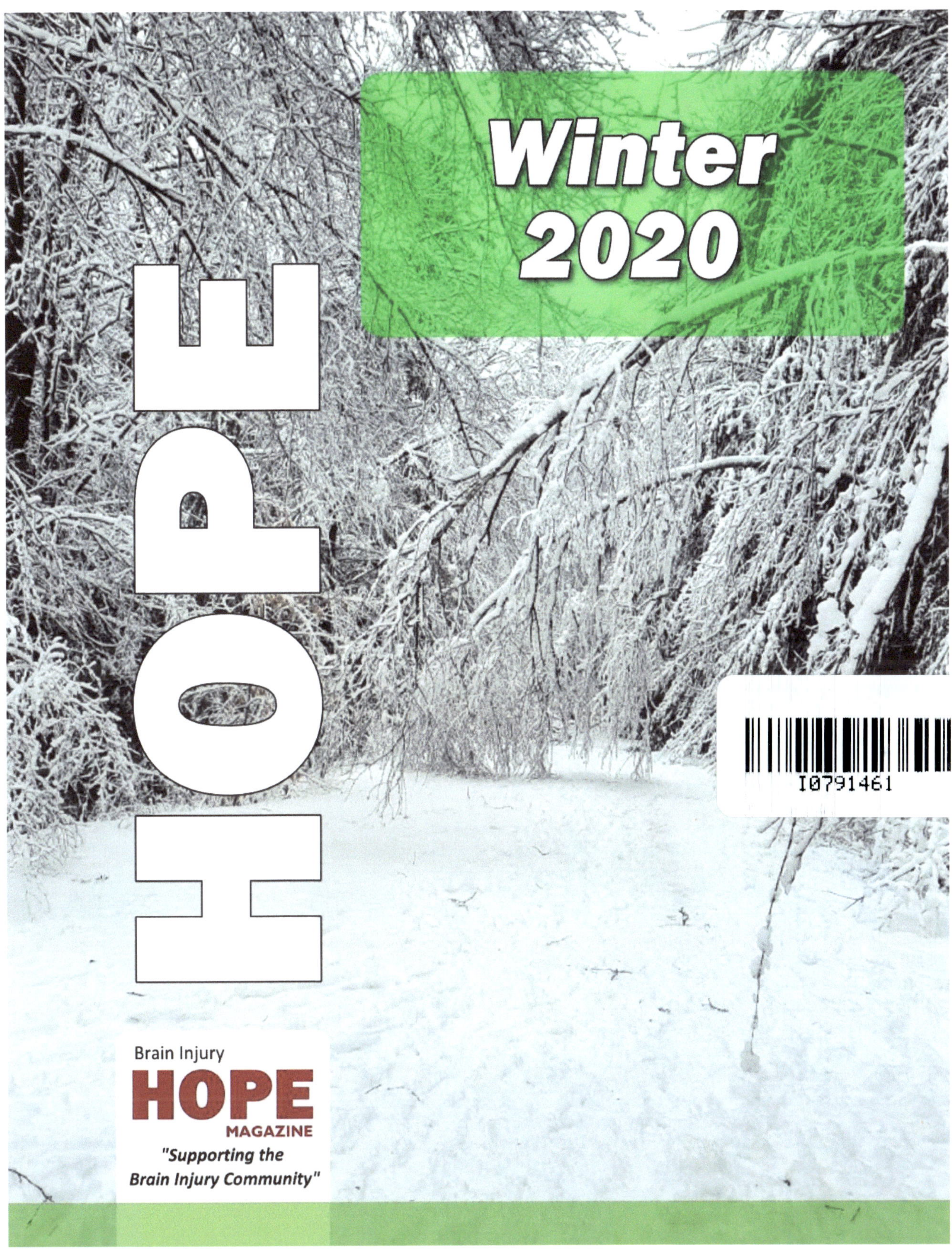

Winter
2020
HOPE
I0791461
Brain Injury
HOPE
MAGAZINE
"Supporting the
Brain Injury Community"

Welcome

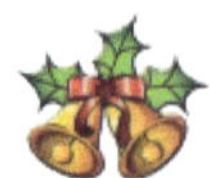

HOPE MAGAZINE

Serving the Brain Injury Community Since 2015

Winter 2020

Publisher
David A. Grant

Editor
Sarah Grant

Our Contributors

Patrick Brigham
Lethan Candlish
Debra Gorman
Sarah Jackson
Lynn Kaye
Peter LeBuhn
Tommy Naudy
Patrick O Callaghan
Nicole Van Vooren
Dr. Sherrill Waddell

Welcome to the Winter 2020 Issue of HOPE Magazine

Join me in taking a deep breath. We have finally reached the end of 2020, a year that will be remembered for so many things. It has been a year of unfathomable loss on so many levels.

Take that deep breath again.

Within the pages of this month's issue, you will find hope, inspiration, and perhaps a bit of distraction for today's troubled world. Like every issue of HOPE Magazine since our 2015 launch, this month's contributors have courageously let us in on their struggles, their hardships, and their hope for a brighter future. We close this month's issue with a firsthand story by our youngest contributor, the ten-year-old of a brain injury survivor.

It's all too easy to get discouraged these days. But for a little while, I invite you to take a break, perhaps pour a cup of tea, and settle down with this month's issue.

Peace,

David A. Grant
Publisher

Table of Contents

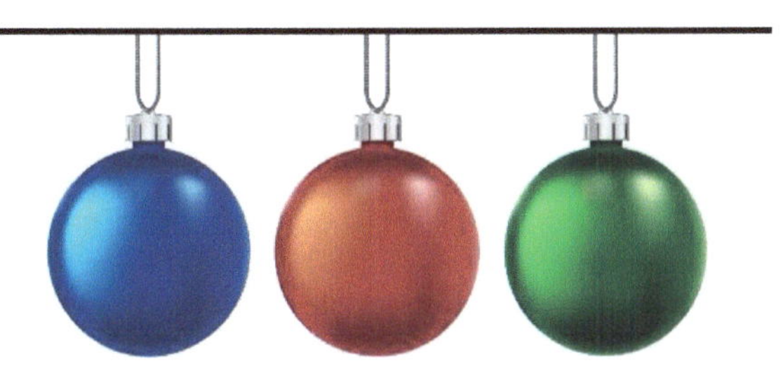

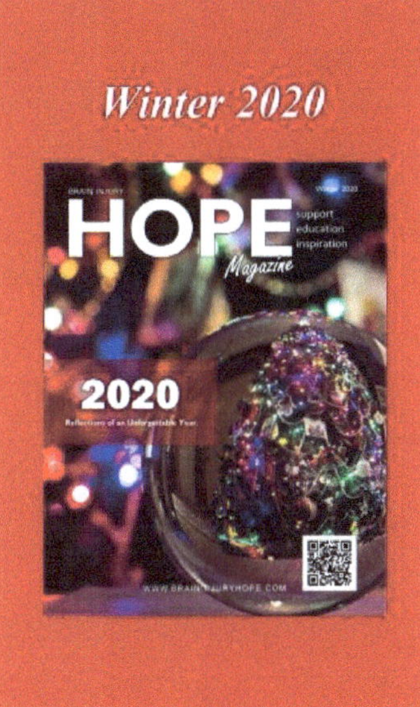

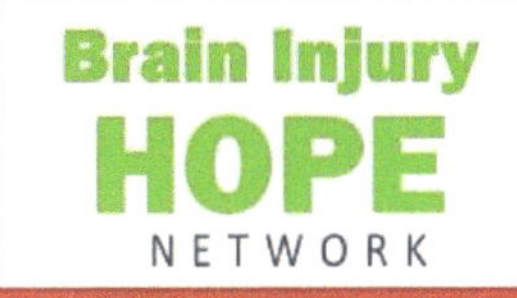

Accepting Responsibility

By Lethan Candlish

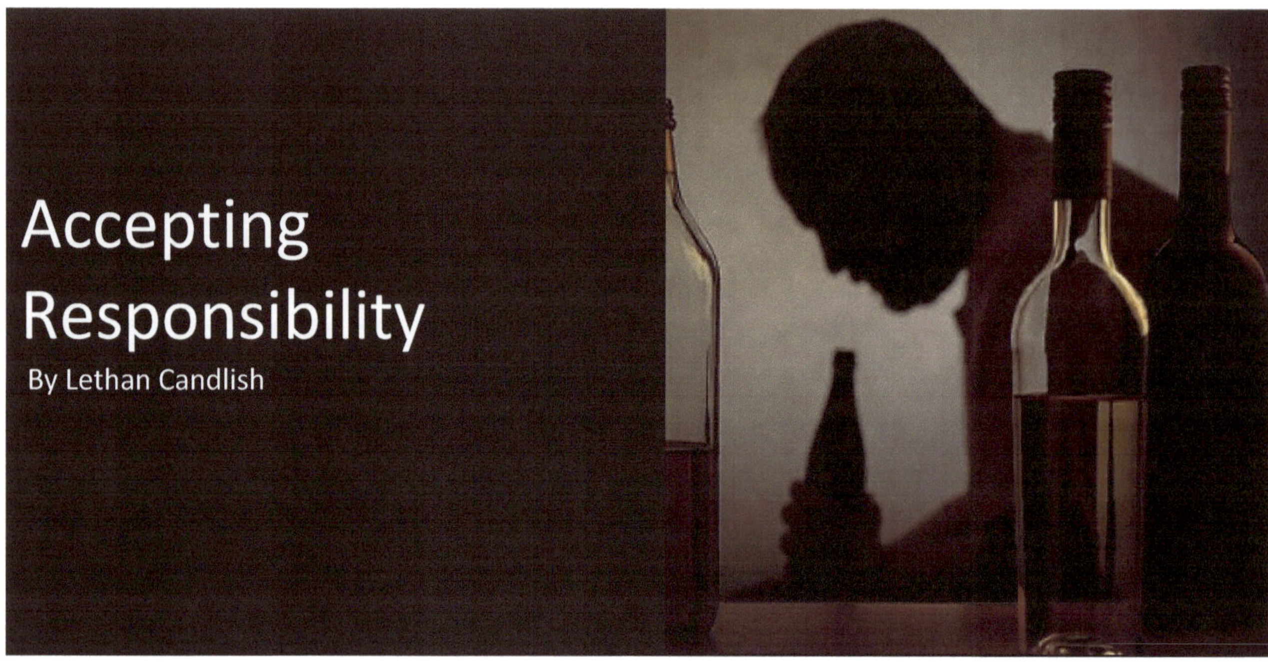

Having a brain injury will affect how a person interacts with the world physically, cognitively, and emotionally. It is also likely that changes in these qualities will contribute to behavioral and social difficulties — at times a survivor may seem ignorant of social conventions or even lash out in a manner that brings physical or emotional pain to those who are close. When such issues arise, it can be tempting for a survivor to blame all such behaviors on "the accident," but this is a dangerous habit. It should be a survivor's goal to return to society without carrying the tag of "brain injury."

Part of that means owning up to one's actions and to not copout of responsibility by using "the injury" as an explanation. In this article, I will present my personal struggle with rage and substance abuse as an example of first avoiding, but then accepting responsibility.

> *"I am a brain injury survivor of fifteen years. After my accident it became apparent that I struggled with both rage and substance abuse."*

I am a brain injury survivor of fifteen years. After my accident it became apparent that I struggled with both rage and substance abuse. I must clarify — when I say, "it became apparent." I mean that other people could see these faults while I refused to acknowledge any responsibility. This struggle could be seen in petulant temper tantrums, drug soaked blacked-out nights, intoxicated rages, emotional and physical destruction, and yet I faulted my injury for all such actions. If there was a problem when I was drugged, I would appear the following morning dressed in what seemed to be appropriate guilt and say, "Hey, look, I'm really sorry. I know I have these issues ever since my injury, and it's not okay that this happens, but I'm really working on trying to stop. I just don't know how to calm this down. It's because of my brain injury, and I'm really trying to fix it. Just know that I know it's not alright."

Yet these words allowed me to believe it was "alright" for fifteen years.

Each time this sheepish apology would fall from my lips, I was lying to myself and to those I had harmed. Perhaps the incident would be forgiven, as my honest eyes and soothing words could at times work rhetorical magic. Sometimes there was simply no more forgiveness and I would be cut off from a lover or friend. When a loss of this sort happened due to some combination of rage and intoxication, I would weep away and damn the accident for cursing me with this burden. In that moment my vow to conquer this "beast of rage" would be renewed, and then I would usually go and get high in order to sooth the pain.

There are mountains of research that show a connection between drug use and rage. I was aware of this, but I was also aware of studies that recognize the tendency for outbursts of violent anger after brain injury. I decided to ignore the first pile of knowledge and focus on the second because the brain injury was what I wanted to be wrong. That way I could persuade myself that I didn't need to stop drugs and alcohol, I just needed to introspectively heal a little bit more. If I could blame my injury, I could ignore the problem, despite a trail of consequences. I lost my place at a university, jobs, friends, lovers, and always I weaseled away when the blame came to me because it was my accident's fault.

Until I lost too much.

A meaningless spat exploded, I drunkenly raged, and the woman I loved and lived with chose her safety and sanity over our relationship. The morning found me hungover on the couch, and she had ended our romance. It was necessary, it was clean, it was over, it was what I would have advised any friend to do.

And it was the unexpected crispness of this consequence that flipped a switch and convinced me to accept responsibility. It didn't matter whether the initiating factor of my anger issues came from the accident or substance abuse. The issue existed and I needed to help myself by getting some help. It was time to try something new and get sober.

As a survivor, it is easy to blame personal faults on brain injury, and it is true that TBI can exaggerate or create less than amiable personality traits, but that cannot be a reason to allow a challenge or flaw to go unaddressed. The injury is an event that happened, but how you live your future is your choice.

If you are a survivor, the physical, mental, and emotional consequences of the injury are now a part of you but should not be how you allow yourself to be defined. In fact, it should be embarrassing to define yourself merely as the product of your tragedy.

You are so much more. Blaming rage on my accident allowed me to hide in an addiction, yet this only amplified the anger I claimed to be trying to fix. It was only after I accepted the flaw of substance abuse as my responsibility that I was truly able to grow.

> **As a survivor, it is easy to blame personal faults on brain injury, and it is true that TBI can exaggerate or create less than amiable personality traits, but that cannot be a reason to allow a challenge or flaw to go unaddressed.**

It's tempting to praise the decision I made to get sober, but it was only the first step in a long path that I am still following. When I made the decision, I had to change friends, locations, and find sources of support for my sober way of life, and this took some time. The romantic relationship I had been in was over because I had behaved inexcusably, yet circumstance and situation conspired to keep my former partner and I working close together.

She saw me make the decision to deal with my anger issues by staying sober, and as time passed a new, different relationship formed in a manner that allows us both to grow. Your actions will be able to change only if you want to be a better person, actively make decisions to foster this new life, and are willing to make an infinite commitment to personal growth.

In my situation, I do still occasionally feel fury begin to swell inside, but now I accept that I must be in charge of my anger and seek to calm it with a sober mind. This struggle with rage and feeling an urge to use drugs will continue all my life, and it may be that these tendencies were amplified by my accident, but now they are a part of me, but just a part of me, not the whole of me. It is my responsibility to ensure they do not take over my life. Brain injury is no excuse for who I am, because I am alive and that gives me a choice of how I show myself to the world.

 My accident happened, but I must allow it to be in my past so that I can flourish as who I am now.

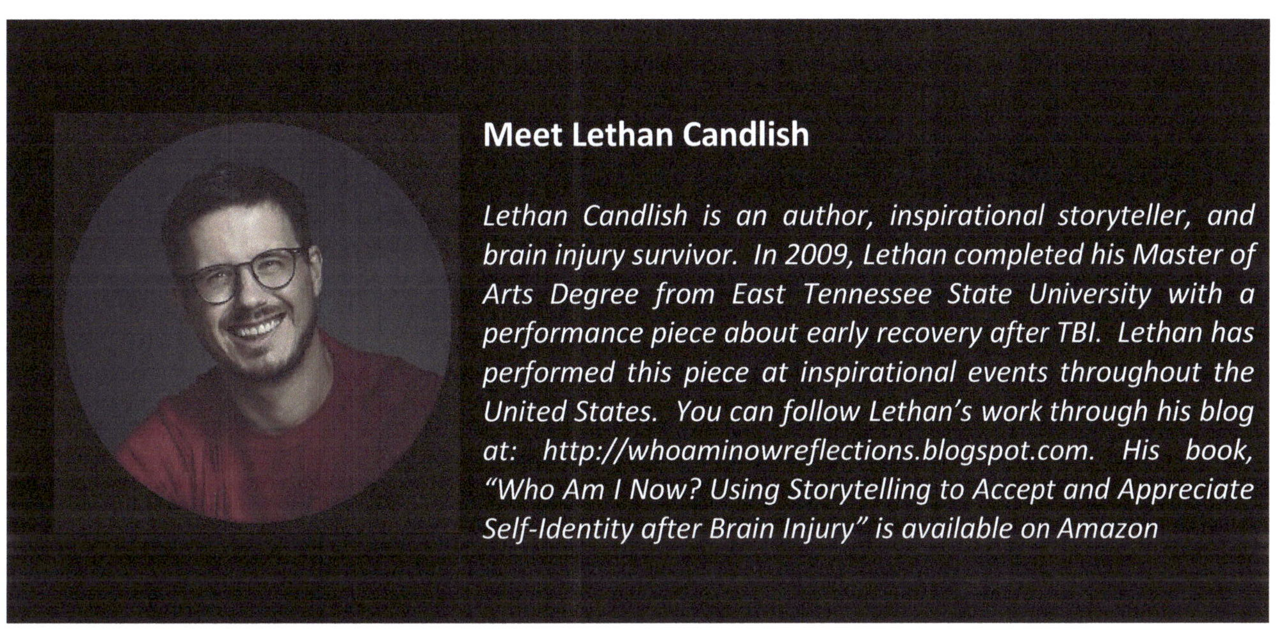

Meet Lethan Candlish

Lethan Candlish is an author, inspirational storyteller, and brain injury survivor. In 2009, Lethan completed his Master of Arts Degree from East Tennessee State University with a performance piece about early recovery after TBI. Lethan has performed this piece at inspirational events throughout the United States. You can follow Lethan's work through his blog at: http://whoaminowreflections.blogspot.com. His book, "Who Am I Now? Using Storytelling to Accept and Appreciate Self-Identity after Brain Injury" is available on Amazon

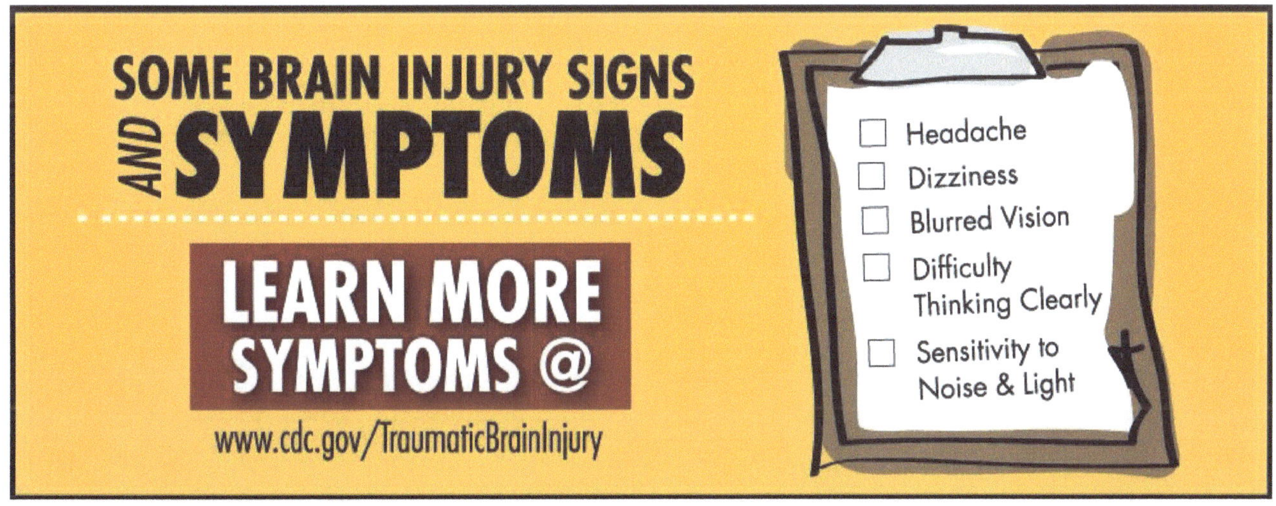

Thinking Outside the Box

By Lynn Kaye

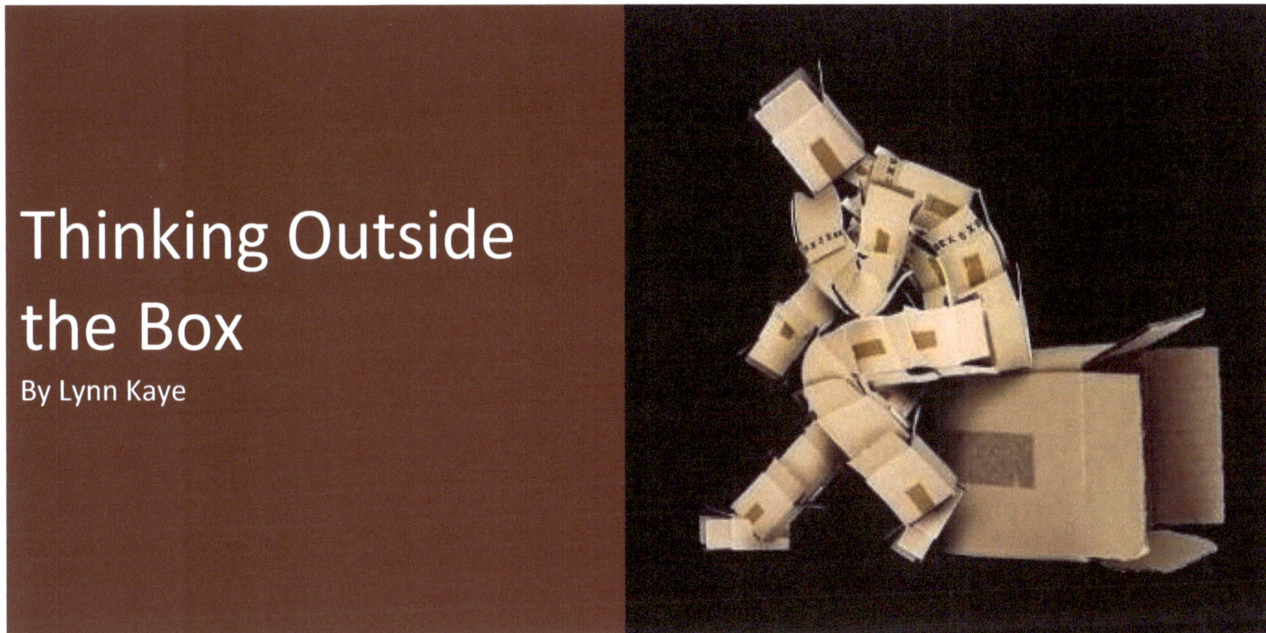

I am a full time caregiver to my husband who suffered an anoxic brain injury in 2011. I have been wanting to write this story for Hope Magazine for a while now, I just never seem to find the uninterrupted time to get my thoughts organized and put on paper.

My husband had a seizure episode on Sunday and is currently hospitalized, unfortunately I cannot be there with him because of Covid-19 visitor restrictions. Hospitals present a huge challenge for my husband because of his visual processing issues, cognitive deficits and right side neglect. I have always been by his side every time. It isn't always easy to be there, but it definitely isn't easy to not be either, waiting for the phone to ring and wondering what is going on. I think of how much harder everything is for him when he is out of his comfort zone.

> *"As I look around our house, I notice everything that has been touched by brain injury and the adjustments that we've made to make this life possible."*

As I look around our house, I notice everything that has been touched by brain injury and the adjustments that we've made to make this life possible. I thought I would share some of the strategies we have developed over the years that keep him fairly independent at home.

We use bright colors to help him see things. Bright red tape is on his car door handle on the inside to help him find it, sometimes he notices it. Bright red tape is also on the side of the bathtub so he can see the side & step over it. We have simplified all of his areas. In his bathroom, only two things are in each drawer so he can tell what they are by feel, not sight. No cleaning supplies under his sink as early on he brought out a bottle of toilet cleaner and asked if it was shampoo. His daily living items have their own place on his bathroom counter, I do not move them, when I clean, I put them back in their spot. He uses bright colored towels & washcloths.

We use bright colored plates so the food may be more noticeable because of the contrast. Bright colored bowls with high sides and curved edges that keep food from falling out and a rubber ring on the bottom that keeps the bowl from sliding around. He does not think to hold the bowl in place.

Using a spoon is almost always easier than a fork because of the vision. For instance, instead of having spaghetti, we have small shell noodles. Most foods are easily adapted to be eaten from the bowl with a spoon. Sharp knives or utensils are hidden so he does not accidentally (or purposely) cut himself. If he spills food or if eating is difficult, he becomes frustrated and angry because it used to be easy and he feels stupid, so I try to make it simple.

Sandwiches are made on hamburger buns. They are smaller than bread and he can hold it with one hand more easily so that nothing falls out. He loves BLT's so I chop everything and mix with the mayo to hold everything together. Bottles of pop and water are used instead of a can or glass as he has a hard time opening a can and may not see it and knock it over. He puts the lid back on the bottles so if knocked over there is no mess.

He has areas of the refrigerator that are his, pop in one spot water in another. Nothing else goes in these areas. I could put rubber bands on the pop so he could tell the different flavors, but he didn't want that. He just drinks whatever one he grabs. Usually he has two choices like Sprite and root beer. They are different color bottles he may pick if he notices the color.

He likes his candy bars cold so there is always a bowl of snack size candy bars in the fridge that are always in the same place.

> "Bottles of pop and water are used instead of a can or glass as he has a hard time opening a can and may not see it and knock it over."

He has his snacks in their place on the counter, either nuts or crackers. So he knows where to find them, I never move them. If I leave something on the counter in his space, he will become confused.

He doesn't prepare any of his own food. I prepare it for him and put it in the designated area where he can easily find it. We use a bright orange bump dot on the microwave so he can feel where the 1 minute button is and heat up his own food.

I put his medications together in a weekly planner and each morning and night I transfer to a pill bottle and put it in the spot where he knows to find it himself so he can take them independently.

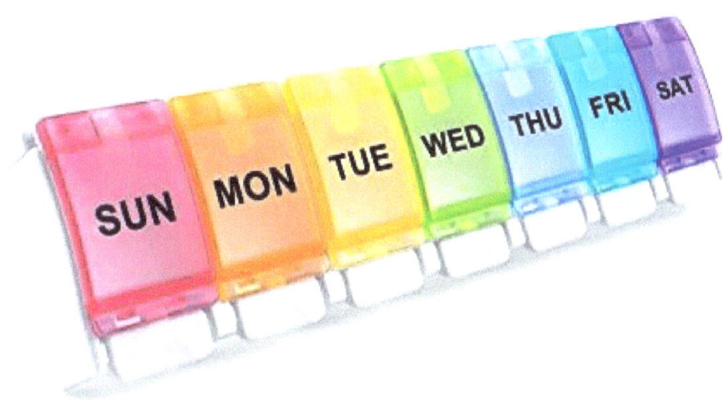

He feeds his service dog himself. I measure out her food and put it into Ziplock baggies along with her daily vitamin. The baggies go into the dog food bin and he grabs a bag and fills her bowl. He would just scoop out a whole bowl full and over feed her if I did not use bags for portion control. Her treats are always in a bowl on top of the fridge. I keep the bowl filled and he can give her treats whenever he wants.

He folds laundry as therapy since it requires him to use both hands. He can no longer bring baskets up from the basement. He only uses the one hand and needs it to hold onto the handrail. He doesn't carry anything on stairs. I bring up the clothes for him and put the white basket by the dark fireplace where he will notice it and fold them when he likes. He usually does the towels and whites. If they are inside-out I fix them before I put them away. He puts the towels away himself, even though they are a little messy, it is great therapy.

He does not like putting socks together anymore since it requires so much coordination. He wears long tube socks because he would put socks on with the heel part on top and then his shoes would not feel right. Tube socks can go in any direction. We switched my socks to ankle length so he could easily tell them apart when he did the laundry. I bought some colored socks for him to have to put the colors together as vision therapy. If he wants a particular sport team shirt, I will find it and hang it on the outside of the closet for him. He has a drawer for socks, a drawer for underwear, a drawer for undershirts and hankies and a drawer for shorts. He knows by the drawer what he has and does not use sight for finding clothes.

He uses electronics for a lot of things. He has three Alexa devices around the house that he uses for the time, news, weather, music, timers, and to set alarms to remind him of things. He also has an iPhone and uses Siri to create notes, text and to call people. He does not use the accessibility feature for the visually impaired because it is too confusing. He keeps his phone on the table in its spot. I put a small piece of Velcro on it so when it rings, he can feel the Velcro and more easily swipe to answer.

He usually does not get to it before it stops ringing so I have assigned all of his contacts special songs when they call so he knows who called him and he can call them back. He has a voice remote for the TV. Anything with buttons is a challenge. He can't feel the different shaped buttons on the remote and can't see them. For a long time, he had a very simple four button remote and I had Velcro on the two buttons he used. I also could change the TV channels from work for him with an app on my phone.

The voice remote we have now has Velcro on the talk button, the OK button and the volume. I'm sure there are other options out there, but this is working for him now and we will stick with it. He loves being able to put movies and shows on himself. He has notes on his phone with his favorite channels. Since he often forgets them, he just asks Siri "what are my notes?"

He enjoys music and has many instruments. He keeps his cowbell, harmonica and tambourine on the end table, his guitar and ocean drum on the lazy boy and bongos on the floor so he can play along to songs on Alexa. He walks on the treadmill. The control buttons were too confusing, so I have it plugged into a power strip. He feels for the switch on that to turn the power on, then he slides the safety switch in all the way.

He helps with the lawn by riding the mower around the back yard. Once he is on the mower all the controls are on the right side. Sometimes he can turn the key by reaching over with his left hand, usually I get it started for him. He only mows the back as he can see the brown fence and that keeps him in our yard. I use the walk behind mower to get the spots he misses.

If he goes anywhere with anyone else, which is very rare, he uses a garage door opener to get in the house, he does not use keys or the keypad code because he does not have the fine motor skills or vision for those. Being somewhere other than home is culture shock for him as he is used to being able to do all these things independently. If we travel, which is hard, he has to rely on me to do more for him.

Public restrooms are a hassle, luckily there are more handicapped ones now so we can go in together as he cannot use one alone. All of these strategies came about by trial and error, thinking outside of the box, simplifying processes, and finding alternative ways to do just about everything. Where there is a will there is a way!

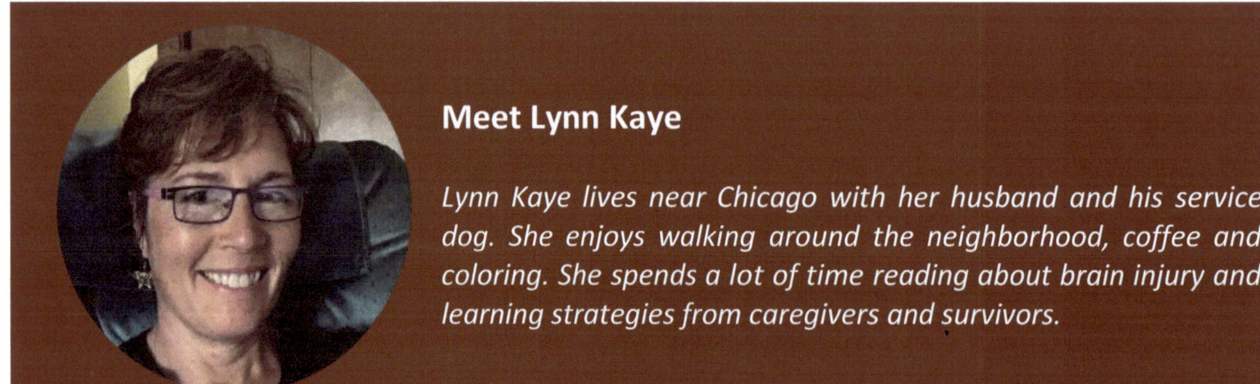

QUIET
EXPLOSIONS
HEALING THE BRAIN
FROM EMMY® AWARD WINNING DIRECTOR JERRI SHER
Traumatic Brain Injury (TBI)
A Silent Killer Impacts
80 Million People
2020
Lilac Award Winner
SpIFF
A FILM ABOUT HOPE & HEALING THAT COULD HELP SOMEONE YOU LOVE
CINEMA LIBRE STUDIO PRESENTS AN EMPIRE PICTURE CORPORATION FILM BY JERRI SHER
INSPIRED BY THE BOOK "TALES FROM THE BLAST FACTORY" BY ADAM MARR & ANDREW MARR PRODUCER JERRI SHER EDITOR ELISA BONORA, ACE
CINEMATOGRAPHER CASEY LYNCH COMPOSER OMRI LAHAV EXECUTIVE PRODUCERS MAGGIE & BILL LYNCH WRITTEN & DIRECTED BY JERRI SHER
CINEMA LIBRE
www.QUIETEXPLOSIONS.com
f /QUIETEXPLOSIONS

Hope From the Wheelchair

By Patrick O Callaghan

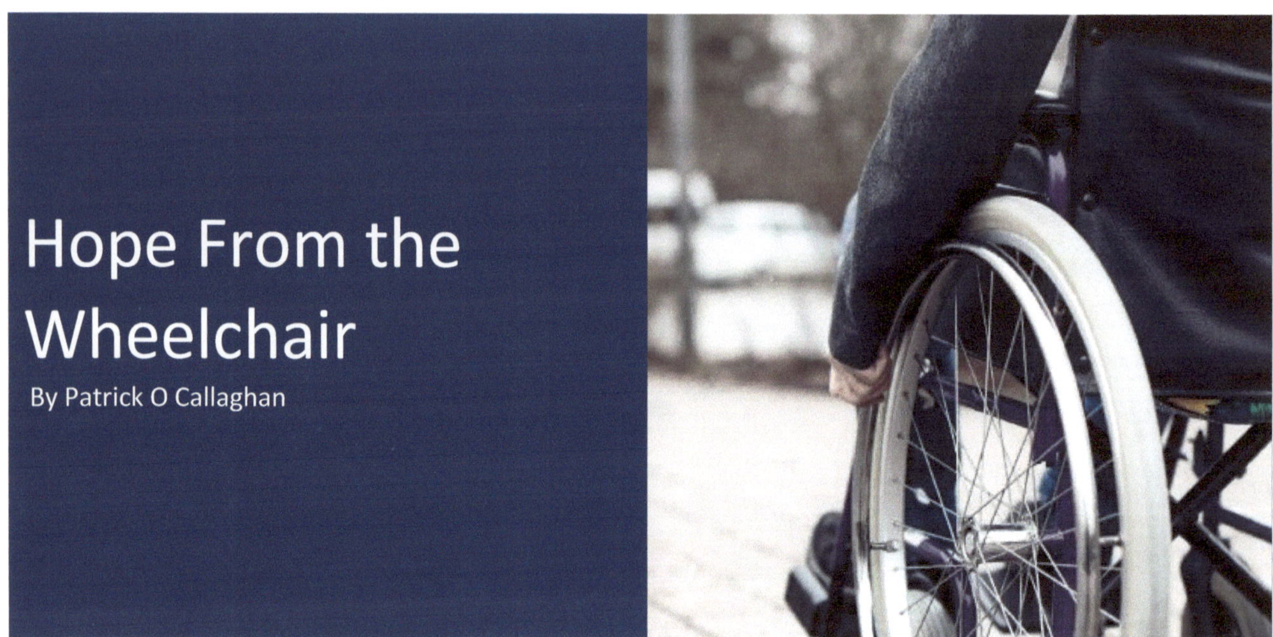

In September 2009, I had the misfortune of falling through a roof while working with my brother, I suffered multiple skull fractures and a compound fracture in my left femur requiring the insertion of a titanium pen. I get about six weeks in the car of University College Hospital in Cork City with a little dental work and most of the fractures finally settling down I was transferred to St. Marys Orthopaedic hospital also in Cork City where I spent a few weeks doing physiotherapy etc. before being sent home for Christmas.

With the help of physiotherapists in south Tipperary general hospitals, the staff in CUH and local services at the age of forty-two I was reasonably mobile again. I was able to enjoy my pastimes of hobby farming and supporting our local GAA football and hurling teams, my three sons being active in both codes.

Throughout this saga, Gillian was steadfastly by my side while paying all of the bills and keeping the aforementioned sons on the straight and narrow, as serious task in its own right.

Alas, Shakespeare's outrageous fortune visited me again in September 2011 while I was out feeding my three pet livestock.

"With the help of physiotherapists in south Tipperary general hospitals, the staff in CUH and local services at the age of forty-two I was reasonably mobile again."

Firstly, I noticed myself to stumble outside of their feeding area but just as my stroke took hold my mobile phone rang in my pocket, it was out second son Riain telling me that he needed a lift because his mother was not home from work. He has always had the best social life in our house.

I told him to find his mother Gillian and my brother Gerry and tell them to come and get me, so I am probably here today because of my mobile phone. When they arrived I had stumbled about 20 metres from where I took the fall, I never remember getting into the car and being taken to the South Doc in

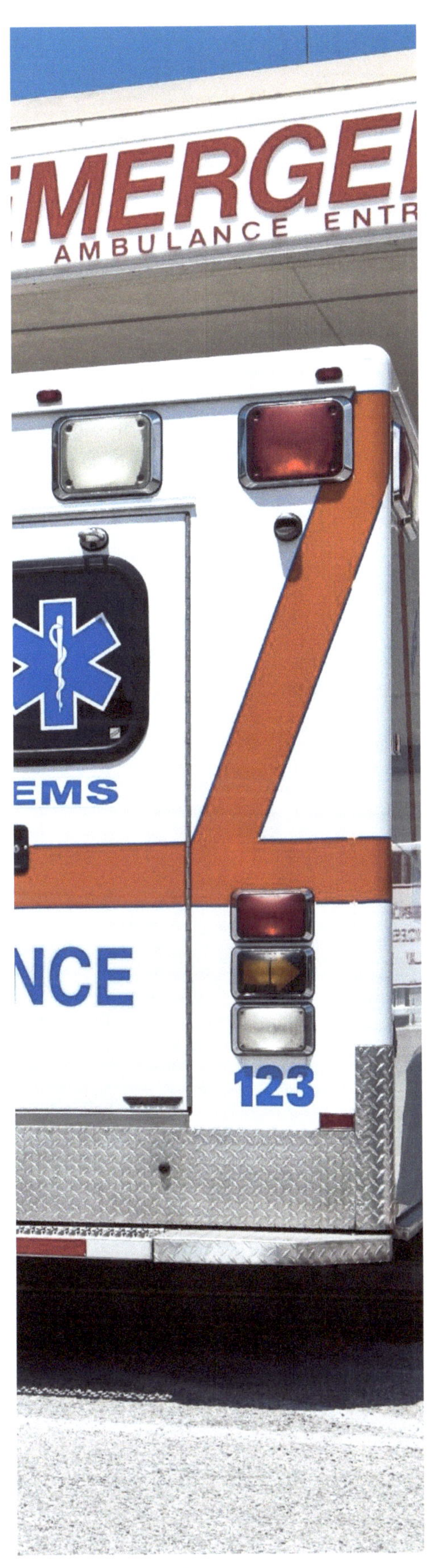

Fermoy Co. Cork – an out of hours service that covers much of North East Cork and South Tipperary, particularly for our of hours emergencies.

On seeing me, the doctor on duty called for an ambulance immediately and I was back on my way to my home away from home, CUH in Cork. In order to relieve brain swelling CUH performed a craniotomy which involved a bone flap being removed from my skull and stored in my groin. Ouch! For the next few days, I was like a cat on a hot tin roof pleading with family and staff members to please take me home.

A week later when I settled down and learned to behave myself I underwent a transoseophogeal from which they discovered that I had an atrial myxoma benign growth in my heart, a particle which had broken off, travelling to my brain causing the stroke. The incidence of this occurring is hundreds of thousands to one and are usually discovered in pathology, trust my numbers to come up on this.

After being operated on to remove the growth from my heart and reinsert the bone flap on my skull I was transferred to the National Rehabilitation Hospital (NRH) in Dublin where I spent over three months hoping to alleviate some of the paralysis on my left side. Unfortunately, the rehabilitative programme in the NRH did not prove to be any way successful, after being fitted with a splint I was sent back home in a very disappointed state of mind.

After being at home for a few weeks and doing exercises on a motomed provided on loan from the HSE shortly thereafter I suffered my first seizure and was taken to south Tipperary general hospital in Clonmel, I spent the month of September there again and when I was eventually released by home, I resumed my exercise regime on motomed.

Nowadays, it has taken each of the intervening years to accept that my life may never get back to where it was before my TBI. It really has been down to my family, friends and the larger community around me that have sustained me through these difficult years. My wife maintained the mortgage whilst keeping our eldest two sons in college, she had to cope with the entire catastrophe, in sickness and health she has always been steadfast and caring regardless of where I was hospitalized it was always a great tonic to see her arrive with our three boys, I'm sure that there were times she wondered which one of us had the stroke (I can be grumpy sometimes – like most men).

My own siblings, all of them along with my parents of the dire straits mantra to a man and woman (they did not desert me my brothers in arms). This was especially true about my brother Jimi who has assisted me with my physiotherapy most evenings over the last seven of eight years.

I do not see my stroke any longer as a sentence, which I did in the earlier years, rather nowadays it is more like a long shadow that I am trying to stay ahead of. Luckily, I am involved with a great support group run by Acquire Brain Injury Ireland in Clonmel Co. Tipperary to which I travel each Wednesday with the option of alternating Thursdays as well. Here about a dozen of us take part in rehabilitative activities that benefit both body and mind. It is very informal setting in which we excel at drinking tea and coffee. We usually start off with our version of mock the week, poking a little fun at whatever politics that are making the national and international headlines of the week.

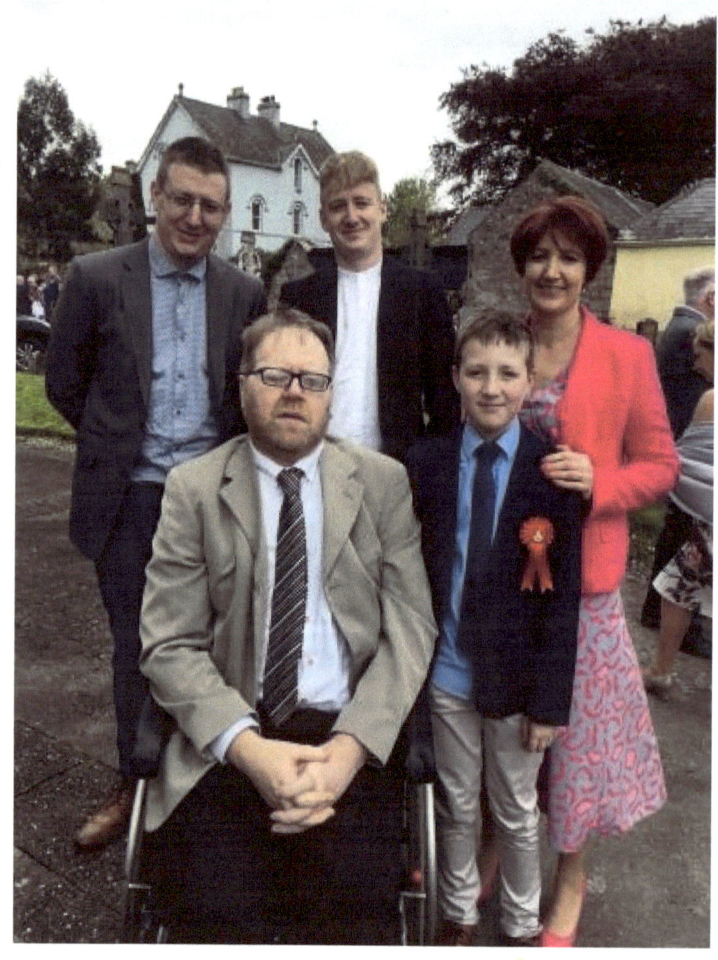

From day one I have struck up some great friendships with so many people, most importantly Matt, Dinah and the two Tommy's, not forgetting Eamonn. Lest I forget whilst outdoors doing a little gardening etc. I can partake in an occasional smoke or two. Probably the biggest mistake a made throughout the entire saga was to return to that terrible habit which destroyed both my teenage and early adult years.

In February of 2012, the aforementioned father went to his eternal reward deservedly, also the second most important woman ever in my life joined him in February of 2016. One of the most annoying aspects of my brain injury was that I was unable to have a meaningful contribution to make in their final years. To anyone out there who finds their lives derailed by the slings and arrows I can only advise you to try and hold onto any little faith you may have in a Devine being, hold onto it as much as possible.

In conclusion, my late mother had some great old Irish phrases; she would have described me as a bit of a mí - ádh (pronounced me – awe) which was her term for a most unlucky person. Even though she suffered from arthritis my mother never lost interest in her family or any of her grandchildren with regards to the inevitability of life. She used to reprimand me even in her eighties by saying to me "nobody likes to go."

Throughout the entire saga to date the most encouraging analysis of my predicament came from our youngest son Rurairí who was five years old at the time, when after being left home for my first Christmas post stroke he accompanied me in to his grandparents' home. Whilst looking at the fire with his hand in his pockets he calmly suggested, "Dad, you can still be alive even when your legs are not working."

> **"Dad, you can still be alive even when your legs are not working."**

Finally, when I wake each morning, I thank the powers - wherever they are - that have allowed me to see another day, but I am determined that one day I will walk again. It will require the use of either a stick or crutch and I am sure it will not be a pretty spectacle (I was never a pretty spectacle anyway- but I still exist.)

By the looks of things when I got on the midnight express of misery I obviously bought a return ticket because I am sitting here today with my left arm in a sling having cracked a bone in my left shoulder and likely to be like this for another month. I managed to topple out of my electric wheelchair while being nosey regarding what was happening in my neighbours' field The wheelchair slipped off an embankment tossing me out onto a hardcore driveway. Murphy's law strikes again!

I must acknowledge the great efforts of all my family, both my children, siblings and in laws and the local community who are so important in fundraising for a wheelchair accessible vehicle, I probably won't live long enough to thank them all properly. I have found over the last nine years that life has gone from sadness to apathy and back to hope. For those of you out there who lead busy lives, do not use the term 'busy' as a reason to neglect having at least one annual check-up in a proper cardiac facility.

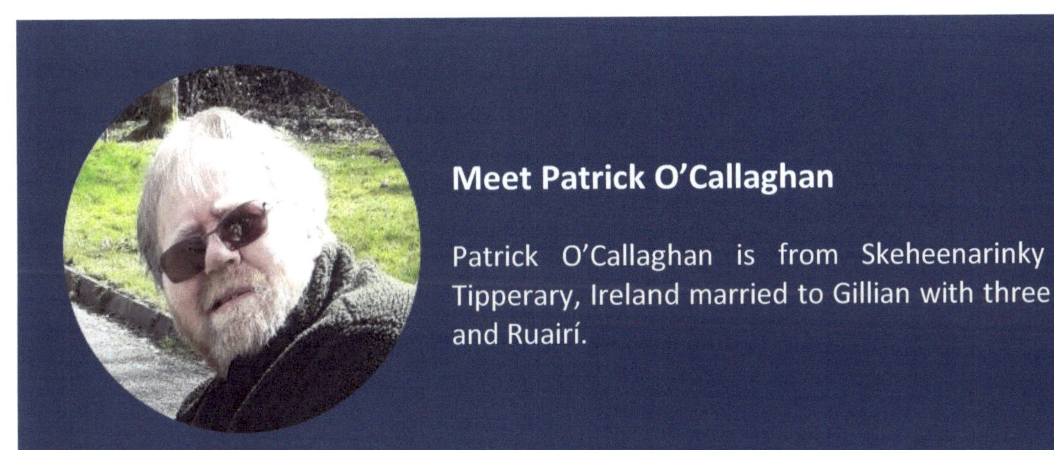

Meet Patrick O'Callaghan

Patrick O'Callaghan is from Skeheenarinky in rural South Tipperary, Ireland married to Gillian with three sons Colm, Riain and Ruairí.

The Pandemic Mom

By Sarah Jackson

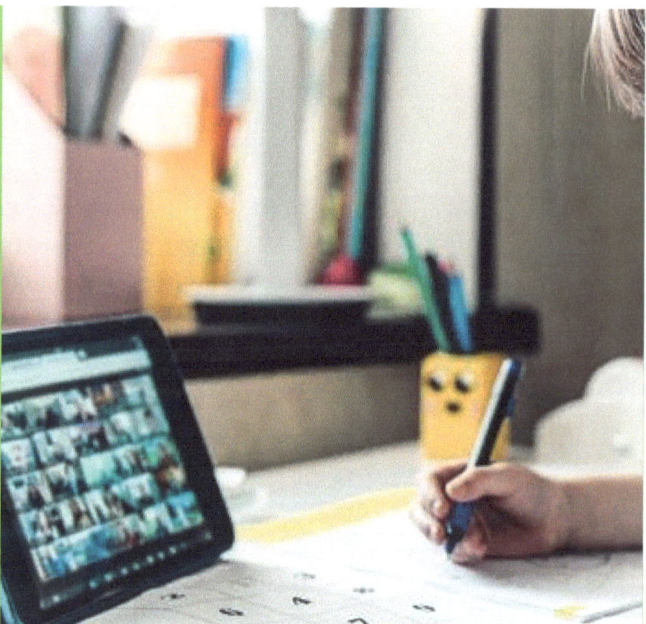

If you're like any other parent these days whose house has become a racetrack, or circus, with two kids, two cats and a dog, you know about the chaos I'm talking about. My email inbox has become overwhelmed, including myself, with mail from teachers and Facebook invites from people I don't even know.

As this new pandemic of virtual and online schooling with meetings and events has swept the nation, I am beginning to think I live inside my computer. Just when I thought I had been doing an impressive job of keeping my kids active and away-from-the-screen, my trusty Lenovo laptop and Apple iPhone informed me they are here to stay. However, kids, as I'm trying to get used to your life now, I think it only fair for you to get used to mine.

> *"As this new pandemic of virtual and online schooling with meetings and events has swept the nation, I am beginning to think I live inside my computer."*

Occasionally, you may see me vacuuming the table in an effort to clean your mess. I haven't gone insane, just utilizing all available tools to help me get the job done quicker. In the morning when you wake up, I may not be here. I have gone for a run, but I'll be home shortly. I have locked the house but either left the keys in the front door or the mailbox, as I don't want to carry them. In the meantime, you can turn the TV on which may be confusing with all those remotes. Instead, you may want to resort to Olivia's Chrome Book, Savannah's tablet in my nightstand (because she stepped on it), my laptop in the kitchen or, if all else fails, a desktop computer downstairs. Now that I think of it, just play with your dolls or wake Dad up.

When I return from my run, I am taking first dibs on the shower. Afterwards, don't be alarmed to see me blow drying my underwear while they are around my waist. I'm just feeling lazy and would rather not turn the dryer on for this single item.

We're going on a picnic today, pack whatever you want. If you want ice cream afterwards, make sure I have my wallet. Make sure I don't put my wallet in the empty lunch bag, then put the lunch bag in the garbage. Trust me: if you don't make this mistake, I will.

We're having meatloaf tonight and surprise, I am cooking. I will be using the electric beaters to avoid dirtying my hands so please step back this time, keep your hands out of the bowl and Vanna, don't plug it in until I tell you to (unless you want a recap of what happened last time).

So, I may not be the "Perfect Mom" but I'm your only Mom. Just as I'm getting used to living with your circus, it would really help if you got used to my circus. As impossible as that is, I still love every moment and day with you. I'll get used to the over-abundance of screen time you need to learn these days, if you get used to the fact that I can be a tad crazy. I'm living with a head injury, a disability and a circus, but I'm making this life work. This life is for you, little one. Don't let anything stand in your way.

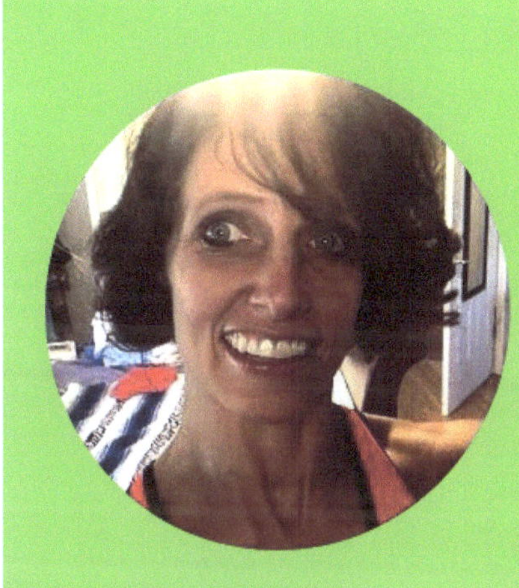

Meet Sarah V. Jackson

Sarah sustained a severe traumatic brain injury at the age of 15 after getting in a car with a underage drinking driver. She is the author of 'You're Getting Better Every Day.' After spreading her story to audiences nationwide, she is now a wife and mother of two girls. Read more about Sarah's story in her book and on her website www.sarahjspeaks.com as she continues to fight the battle of drinking and driving, underage drinking, poor choices and traumatic brain injury awareness.

Living With Hope

By Patrick Brigham

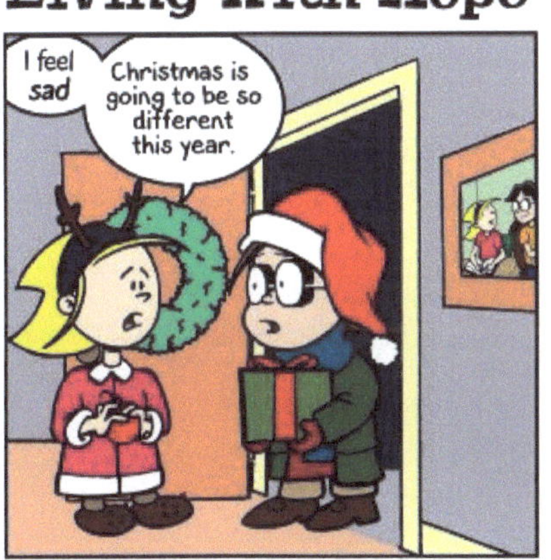

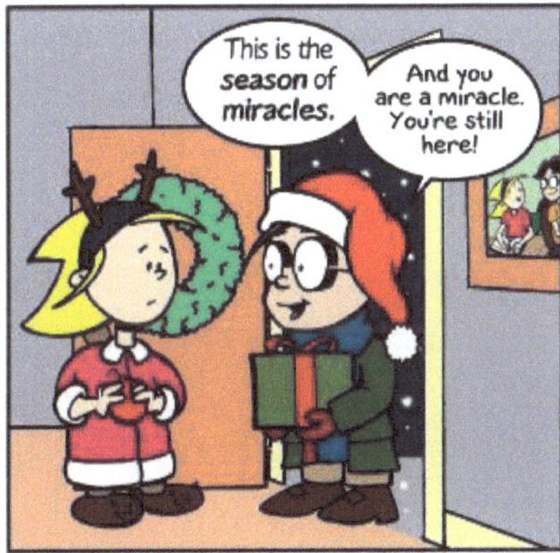

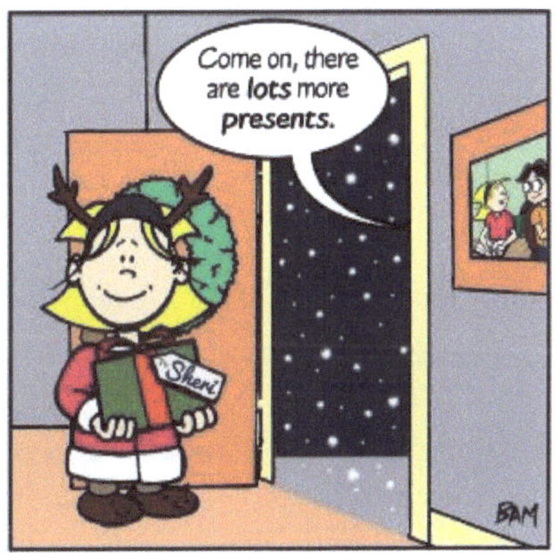

5,716 Days

By Debra Gorman

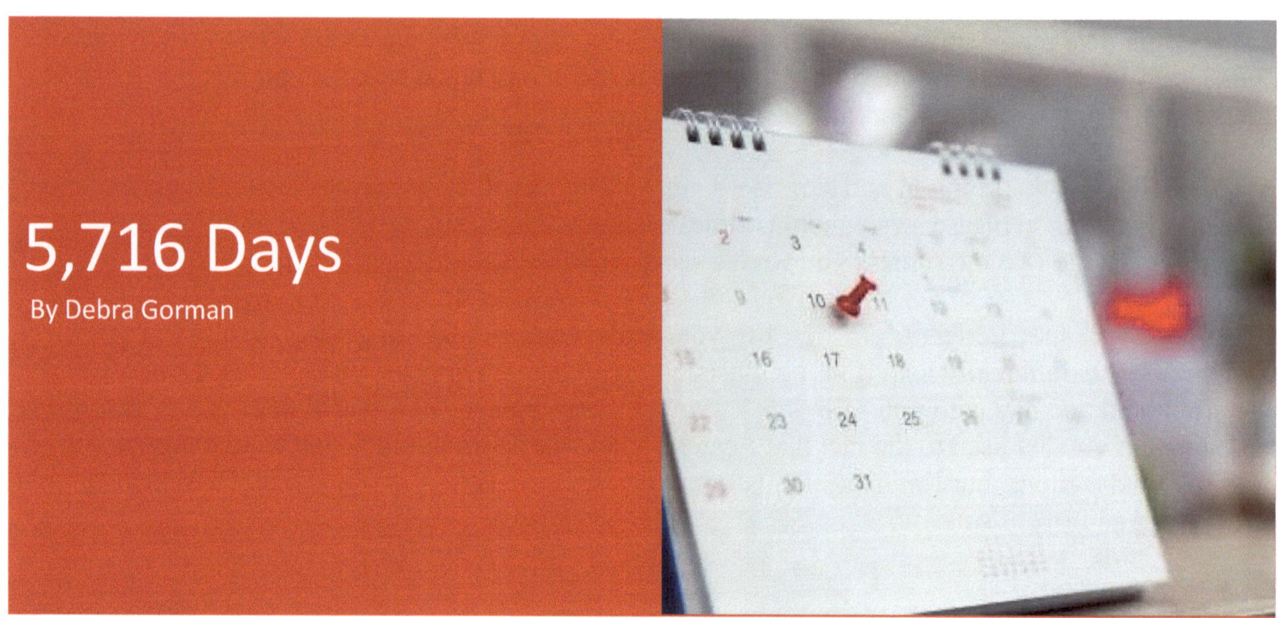

Every year for nearly a decade I have commemorated the date, August 20th. It's not my actual birthday, nor is it our wedding anniversary. It's both a birthday and an anniversary, though. August 20, 2011 is the day I didn't die.

It is the anniversary of the brain hemorrhage that nearly took my life. I got a do-over that day. There is plenty I don't like about my present physical condition, but I am determined to make the most of the days I have left, because I'm convinced I'm still here for a reason, and I want to fulfill my mission.

I learned that the average woman lives to be 81 years old. I do not see myself living that long. Let's say I do live to be 81, that's 16 years from now, 5,716 days at the time of this writing. I want to live each day that I am given with intention. If I am blessed enough to live even one more day, I hope to be a blessing to someone else. And I want to enjoy the time I have left. I believe that being here means I have more to do. I am also convinced I have the ability to *choose* joy, although sometimes it takes conscious effort. There have been times I thought I would collapse from the exertion. That is what I mean by living intentionally. There is no point in waiting until all the hard stuff is behind me. That will never happen.

"If I am blessed enough to live even one more day, I hope to be a blessing to someone else. And I want to enjoy the time I have left."

I read a quote recently that I want to be my life's motto: *"Life isn't about waiting for the storm to pass, it's about learning how to dance in the rain."* Think about that. Isn't that a great quote? You may think it is simplistic, but profound truths are usually simple. Storms will come, bad things will happen. To learn be joyful in spite of difficult circumstances is the goal. It makes me think of that movie from 1952 with Gene Kelly and Debbie Reynolds, *Singing in the Rain.*

Bon Jovi had a particular hit, released May 23, 2000. Sometime after that, it became an anthem, of sorts, for me. Every weekday morning, I would hear the song on the radio as I drove to college. It wasn't out of my way to drop my daughter off at her school, so she was usually with me when the song came on the radio and I cranked up the volume. On cue, she would roll her eyes as I started to sing with the band. The lyrics of the chorus deeply affected me every single time I heard the song:

It's my life
It's now or never
I ain't gonna live forever
I just want to live while I'm alive.

I had no idea how those words would continue to affect me even a couple decades later. At the time the song meant a lot to me because I was doing something that felt bold. I was going to college in my late forties. I was raising my three daughters and working nearly full time. I felt fully and meaningfully alive, although I had chosen a difficult path. I could say the same thing today, only this time the path chose me.

I assume we all feel limitations. I see those limitations as brackets, or parenthesis, which often contain something special. We may be able to serve humanity in ways we have never considered before, ways that only we can, because of our hurtful experience.

"I assume we all feel limitations. I see those limitations as brackets, or parenthesis, which often contain something special."

Long before my brain bled, I saw the value of celebrating milestones, of celebrating life. Celebrations reflect gratitude. They place a mental bookmark to remind us to remember. While it's true my life looks different than before the brain bleed, I try to remember I'm no less valuable or worthy.

Over the years I have commemorated August 20th in various ways. In the past I have invited friends over for a butterfly release party. One year my husband and I sat on our patio, talked about life and released balloons into the early evening sky. This year we went on a picnic on a nearby mountaintop. Later, we went for ice cream with our pup. Writing this is also part of the commemoration.

I encourage all of us to remember that if we're breathing, we belong here and we have purpose. It will not be easy. We will make mistakes. Sometimes we'll feel heroic just to make it through the day. And that will be true. On those days, maybe especially on those days, let's remember when our head hits the pillow to say thank you. "Thank you" can be a prayer that says we appreciate the ability to close the book on another day. Sometimes that will be enough.

Most days let's sing loudly, and with boldness, "I just want to live while I'm alive".

While it's true my life looks different than before the brain bleed, I try to remember I'm no less valuable or worthy.

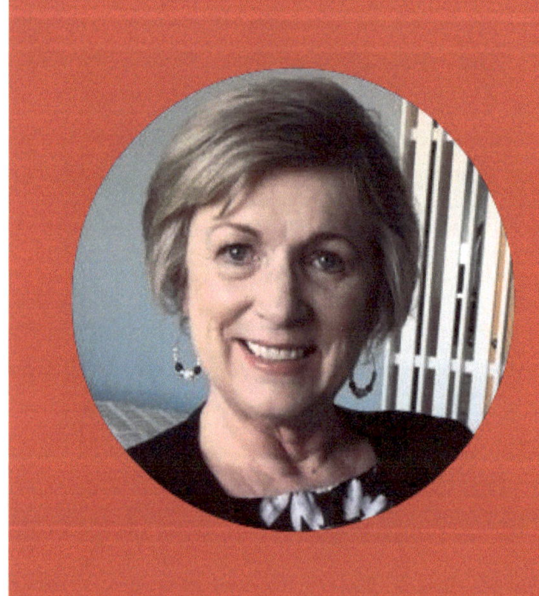

Meet Debra Gorman

Debra Gorman was fifty-six years old in 2011 when she experienced a cavernous angioma on her brain stem, causing her brain to bleed. Four months later she sustained a subdural hematoma. In the blink of an eye life became very different. She lacks the balance and coordination to do any of those activities. Debra finds a creative outlet in writing. She enjoys writing for her children and grandchildren and has written articles that have been published for hospice. Currently, she writes for her blog, entitled Graceful Journey. Read more at debralynn48.wordpress.com.

The TBI Cascading Effect

By Dr. Sherrill Waddell

A cascade is water falling from a high point in the landscape making its way down steep slopes in stages until it smoothens out in a pool on the bottom. This natural marvel, cascading from a high point to a low point, is used to describe the residual effects of Traumatic Brain Injury (TBI). Research discusses the cascading effect related to the impact on neurodegeneration and the physiological component regarding the decline that takes place within the brain. There is an equivalent diminishing factor to this matter with TBI as well.

"The number of close friends and family members became fewer, some by their choice and others by mine."

Survivors face the daunting task of living a life drastically altered from the one they knew. Not only do they face a cascading effect with an increased rate of cognitive decline, but endure a torrent of uncontrollable, forced upon life changes as the survivor deals with the many challenges of the diagnosis in several areas of life. The initial injury is just the catalyst for a chain of life events that are not welcomed or even comprehensible for people unfamiliar with TBI.

People diagnosed with a brain injury have to deal with head trauma and several other aspects of life that drastically change. For many, such as myself, life contracted with a TBI diagnosis. It is the result of instinctual survival skills that kick in to save brain energy. The number of close friends and family members became fewer, some by their choice and others by mine. Career titles were replaced with medical acronyms and components of my life I had purposely chosen were instantly wisped-away as I was forced to live a life that I would not have chosen. Instead of working and sharing experiences with coworkers, I found myself going to appointments where I was continually poked and prodded and evaluated. Overall, the inner and outer circles of people I interacted with ebbed in and became smaller without my consent or my permission.

Additionally, there is an entire spectrum of how TBI survivors can handle their emotions after the injury. Some become angry and bitter and unleash that harshness on the world around them. Many become depressed and develop anxiety. Others are able to cope with the changes in a somewhat manageable manner. I have found myself on any point of the spectrum of the wide range of emotions as I've tried to maneuver through the life changes that have taken place. The emotional component of being forced to live completely different than the life lived pre-TBI diagnosis is a challenging journey both for the survivor and those who knew him or her before.

The TBI cascading effect may cause debility in many areas of a survivor's life, such as the social and emotional parts mentioned above. Personally, the number of my close relationships are smaller, but they are more meaningful. Additionally, being instantly confronted with lability sent me on journey inward towards reflecting on what I really wanted out of life and accepting the person I truly was after my injury as well as who I still wanted to become. I was told that the most significant gains occur during the first year repeatedly throughout rehab. It is almost as if the medical world verbally prescribed a script indicating the TBI cascading effect would continually occur and life would be downhill after the one-year mark.

Looking back over the past seven years, this is not the case. I have continually challenged myself not only in the fight to stay alive but in deciding what kind of life I want to live. I have stopped feeling as if my TBI diagnosis dictates who I am and directs what I do on a daily basis. Instead, I have chosen to live life according to what I enjoy doing and make choices that lead me to contentment and fulfillment.

Personally, the number of my close relationships are smaller, but they are more meaningful.

Meet Dr. Sherrill Waddell

Dr. Sherrill Waddell is a traumatic brain injury survivor, an adventurer, mother, sister, aunt, and friend. She currently lives in Florida and enjoys long walks in nature, reading, writing, and spending time with her animals and her family and friends. She also enjoys traveling to National Parks all over the world and is working on writing a book about her experiences in these wild spaces. She is working on sharing her journey to recovery and seeing how she can help those going through this incredibly difficult challenge.

There Are Always Things You Can Do!

By Peter LeBuhn

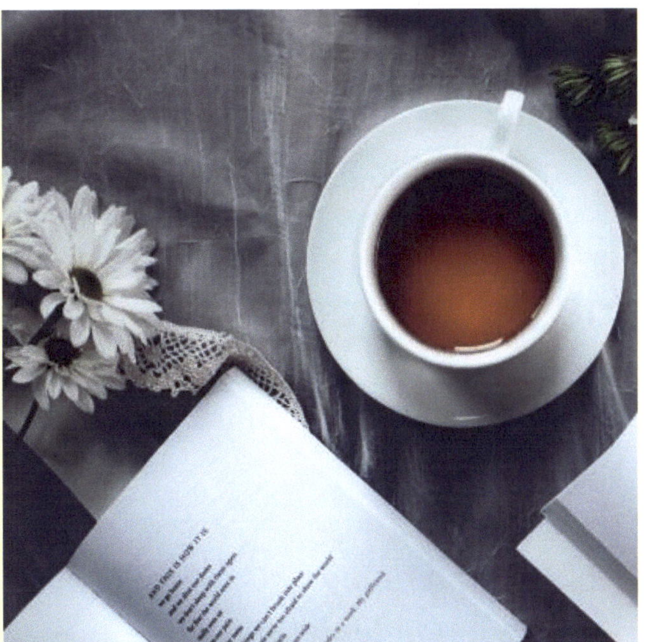

I was born on February 21st, 1964. My father walked in from work and he said to my mom, Jeanne, "What is for dinner?" She said, "Honey it is time." He said, "Oh good because I am hungry." Mom said "Not that time. We are going to have our child soon." I was born thirty-eight minutes later.

At the age of six months, I had a medical emergency that almost ended my life. I was put in a tub of ice to cool my body temperature. It was 107. I had my first seizure at age four and have dealt with epilepsy and subsequent traumatic brain injury for my entire life.

I have lived a lifetime of seizures and challenges. All I have ever known is a life with epilepsy, so I learned to adapt to different situations. I have had to give up different parts of my life like driving, living independently, drinking the amount of fluids I want, playing sports, etc.

> *"I had my first seizure at age four and have dealt with epilepsy and subsequent traumatic brain injury for my entire life."*

Having these issues made me have to look outside myself and try to help other individuals. I have written a poem that I would like to share. The poem is called Electrical Storm and it is my gift to you.

Electrical Storm

Living a life that is sunny
Walking around
I am happy
Now feeling funny
What is going on
What is happening
An electrical storm
A party is going off in my brain
One that I cannot explain
Don't like this party
Don't want to be here
Living in fear
This is no way to live
Living a life with a light on my heart
Thy life from here will make my start.
A start of sharing and caring.

When I was younger, my mother, family and I could have hidden away from life, but we chose not to. We were an example to others. We moved to Pennsylvania when I was nine years of age. My mother searched for a group that would support parents of children who have brain disorders.

She met a well-known real estate agent at the time who had a daughter with the same disorder as I have. They began meetings and started a foundation with Jefferson Hospital in Philadelphia and now there are many branches of the foundation across the United States.

And to think it all started in a living room that grew into an international foundation to helps individuals. It is now called Epilepsy Foundation Eastern Pennsylvania. We needed to figure out a way to make money, so we got creative.

We made money through strolls and fundraisers. We started in 1976. We began going to Philadelphia Phillies games at Veteran's Stadium and some of the ticket cost would go to our foundation.

We also did a Mardi Gras dinner each February to raise money. We had a band and former Miss America winners attended. Mayors of the City attended. The foundation still has an annual Mardi Gras fundraiser.

The foundation helps spread awareness about epilepsy and it helps the individuals and families have a support system. It's important to focus on what you can do for someone else or a group rather than what you cannot do. So that's what I did.

I began writing in eighth grade. I was a good friend with my English teacher. In the summer my family went to Iowa on our family trip. I wrote her a letter and I got it back with lots of corrections. I was offended because nobody ever corrected me in a letter before but I'm glad because it motivated me to do better in English.

In fact, I was an English major in college and went on to write poetry books including *Writing From the Spirit* and *Poems From the Heart*. My books can be bought on Amazon and my poems are also viewable at www.poemhunter.com/peter-lebuhn.

I try to be a good example to everyone. No matter what situation you are in, there are always things you CAN do.

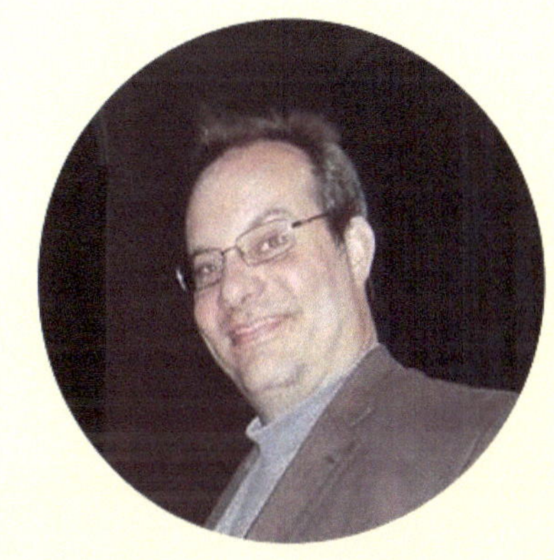

Meet Peter LeBuhn

Peter Lebuhn is a 56 year old man who currently lives in Malvern, PA at a group home with other people who have traumatic brain injuries. He has been through lots in his life and has accomplished many things. He hopes to inspire others with his story.

Always turn a negative situation into a positive situation.

— *Michael Jordan*

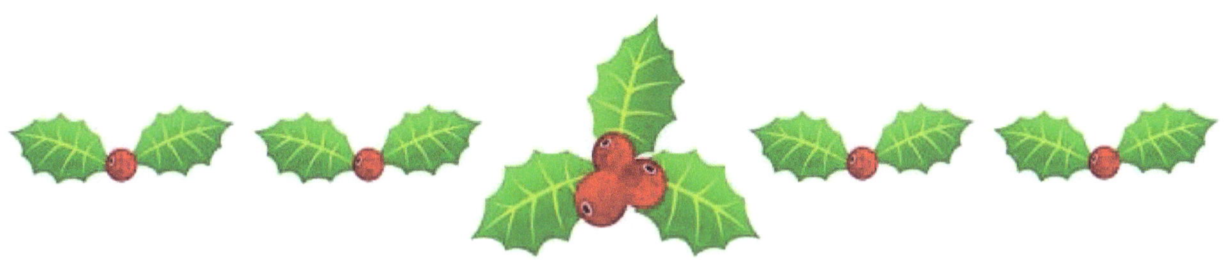

A World Turned Upside Down

By Nicole Van Vooren

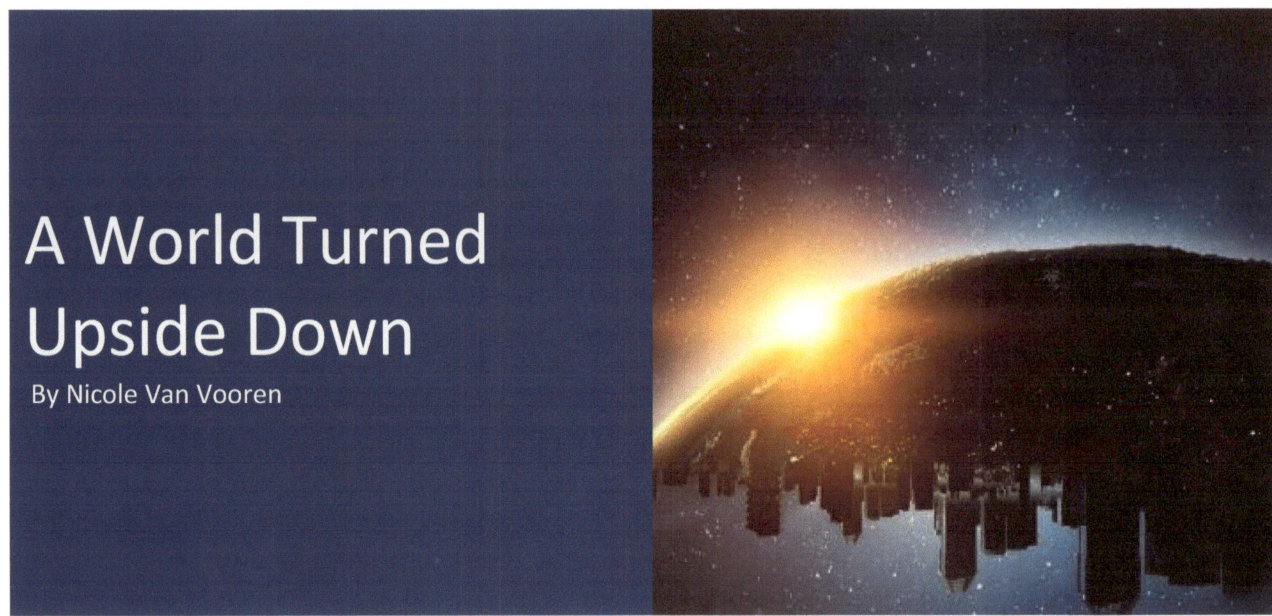

I found myself looking in the mirror of the hospital bathroom and asking myself what is going on? That was the day that I realized that my life had changed forever. I was so confused not knowing anything. Where I was, what day it was, who I was with. Everything seemed to be so confusing. I started crying and screaming I didn't know what to do. I didn't understand anything that was going on. I felt like a different person. I felt completely empty inside.

My parents sat with me and tried explaining to me what had happened. They told me I had a brain tumor that was cancerous, and I almost died. They told me that they had to remove a large tumor that was located in the frontal lobe of my brain. I couldn't understand anything. I kept asking myself how this is happening to me? I was completely fine. I was having, a very difficult time grasping even the smallest concepts, or easily forget them.

> *"My parents sat with me and tried explaining to me what had happened. They told me I had a brain tumor that was cancerous, and I almost died."*

After spending a month in the hospital all I wanted was to go home. The day I went home I was so happy, but my struggles began. I couldn't play outside, watch tv and understand it. I would get terrible headaches and seizures. I would constantly get mad, sad, frustrated, I couldn't control my emotions. I felt like a light switch one second I was fine and the other second, I exploded for no reason.

My parents tried being so supportive and helping me as much as they could. They were always by my side. The wanted me to be as normal as I could. The problem wasthat I couldn't, I wasn't the same person anymore. I had lost my identify. Everything became a struggle. Going to school was miserable I became very depressed. Kids in my class would torture me because they said I looked like a Monster. I was overweight because of all the medication I was taking and had no hair, I was constantly bullied. That's when I developed an eating disorder. I never ate or I was always throwing up. I didn't want to be made fun of anymore.

I was labeled as the monster every time kids saw me, they said I belong to a Halloween movie. I was never invited to birthday parties or play dates because they said they were scared the way I looked. I became very lonely and didn't talk to anyone. As I got older my struggles became even more noticeable. I wouldn't fit in because my mentality was of a child. I wanted to play with dolls, play with my stuff animals, and watch Disney movies.

At this point I had no friends. My brother and sister tried being part of my life, but I also pushed them away. I had terrible behavioral problems. It was very hard for me to control my temper. There were times that I would get so frustrated that I would bite myself, cut myself, hit myself. I didn't know how to control my emotions. The harder I tried in school the worse I did. Nothing came easy to me anymore. I had to study for hours to get barely pass a class. I was so frustrated because I knew that my dreams of becoming a doctor were getting harder and harder to reach.

When I got into high school, I wanted to fit in. I started taking acting classes. They taught me how to walk, talk, and act. I started focusing on my body, my eating disorder got worse. All I wanted was to be normal, but my life got worse. I was very bad at making decisions, so I started getting taken advantage of. I was very easily manipulated by everyone because I had a very difficult time understanding right from wrong. I struggled so much that I became suicidal. I couldn't stand leaving this way anymore.

The biggest struggle was trying to make people understand that I had a disability, but it wasn't visible. I was constantly discriminated and to this day it still happens to me.

Every time I ask someone to repeat themselves or for help, they get offended. I have told people several times that I'm disabled but there answer to me is you look normal. This has been extremely difficult for me. I have accepted that I have a disability, but it is not easy. I'm married to a great guy. I have two boys a nine-year-old and a 1thirteen-month-old.

There are still days that I wake up not knowing where I am. It is very difficult to struggle so much doing the most basic task. Sometimes I yell and get into an argument with my husband for no reason. I have such a hard time controlling my emotions because they are all over the place. I'm also extremely frustrated because I was never able to accomplish my dreams. There days I don't know why I'm still alive, but I remind myself that I'm still here for a reason Living like this can be very challenging.

I'm always very tired, and I suffer from terrible headaches. Some days are better than others. My nine-year-old son is my hero he has been there by myside helping me regardless. And my little guy keeps me going every day. I wouldn't be able to continue living with all the struggles if it wasn't for all the support I have from my husband and my family.

There are still days that I wake up not knowing where I am. It is very difficult to struggle so much doing the most basic task.

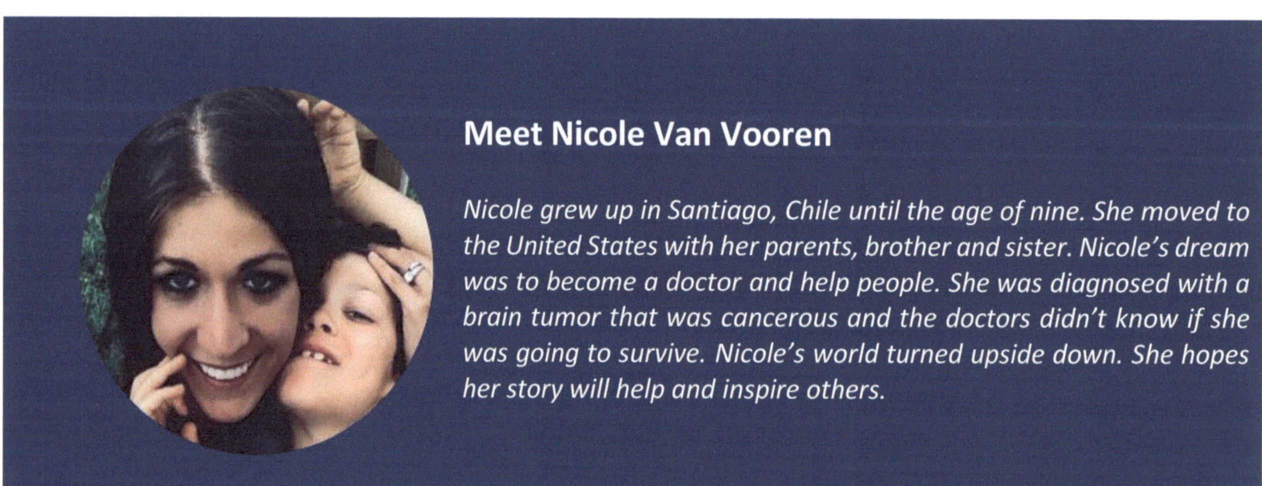

Meet Nicole Van Vooren

Nicole grew up in Santiago, Chile until the age of nine. She moved to the United States with her parents, brother and sister. Nicole's dream was to become a doctor and help people. She was diagnosed with a brain tumor that was cancerous and the doctors didn't know if she was going to survive. Nicole's world turned upside down. She hopes her story will help and inspire others.

Courage doesn't always roar. Sometimes courage is the quiet voice at the end of the day saying 'I will try again tomorrow.

-Mary Anne Radmacher

Mommy's Brain Injury

By Thomas Naudy

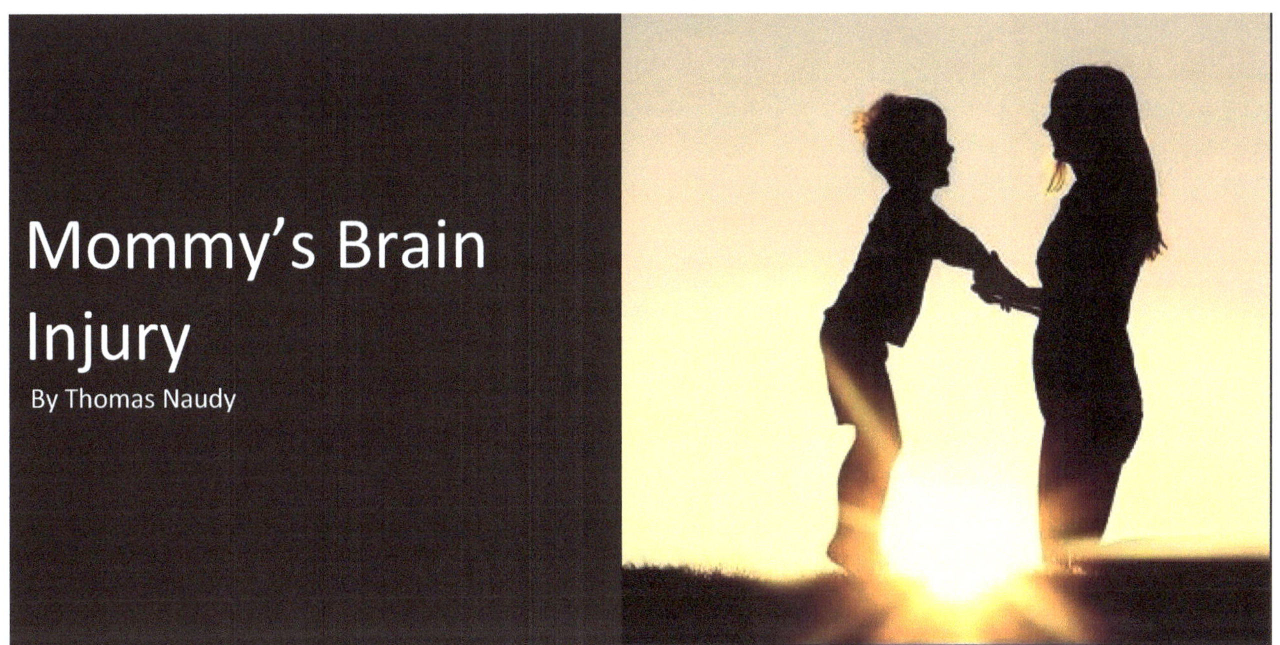

My name is Tommy I'm nine years old. I'm currently in fourth grade. My Mommy is a survivor of a traumatic brain injury. She was diagnosed with a brain tumor that was cancerous. The tumor was located in the frontal lobe of her brain. The doctors thought that my mommy was going to die. My mommy survived because she fought so hard. The size of her tumor was the size of a tennis ball. She had her surgery done in Westchester Medical Center.

My mom was left with many problems. Having that part of her brain removed caused her emotions to be all over the place. She gets mad very easily, she also gets very frustrated when she can't perform an easy task, that happens very often. Sometimes she cries because she gets sad for no reason. She also has problems with her memory, she is always forgetting where she puts things, to call her doctors, to eat and sometimes to even drink water.

"Since I was a little boy I have always seen mommy struggle in many ways. She has always been there by my side and tried being the best parent she could."

She forgets when I show her things over and over. She has a very hard time with loud noises and has very bad anxiety. My mommy doesn't like being around crowds of people. Many people have been mean to her and hurt her because she doesn't understand. The hardest part for my mommy is that she looks normal and everyone doesn't believe she struggles and has a traumatic brain injury but my mommy was left mentally challenged.

Since I was a little boy I have always seen mommy struggle in many ways. She has always been there by my side and tried being the best parent she could. She is always playing with me. I always take lots of pictures so when she forgets I can show her and remind her how much fun we had. It has been very hard for me to have a disabled parent. I wish she was normal and didn't forget so much. It makes me very sad, but I am also very happy because she is very kind to me and has taught me so many things that I would have never known with out her. This has made me really strong there has been many times that I have been away from my mommy because she had to go to hospitals to get better. I hate when my mommy leaves me, but I have always gone to visit her and this has made me into a better person.

My dream is to become a brain surgeon, and help people that go through this. I don't like when people make fun of anyone with a disability it makes me very sad and mad. People don't choose to have a disability. I have always been very lonely because nobody understands me, kids can be very mean because I'm different I rather read books about anatomy and biology than play video games. I also love spending time with my mommy.

> # My dream is to become a brain surgeon, and help people that go through this.

My goal in life is to study really hard and get into the best medical school. I love to help people by donating toys and food to charity. I hope that one day I can achieve my dream and travel around the world doing brain surgeries for free for people that are poor. I want to save as many lives as I can.

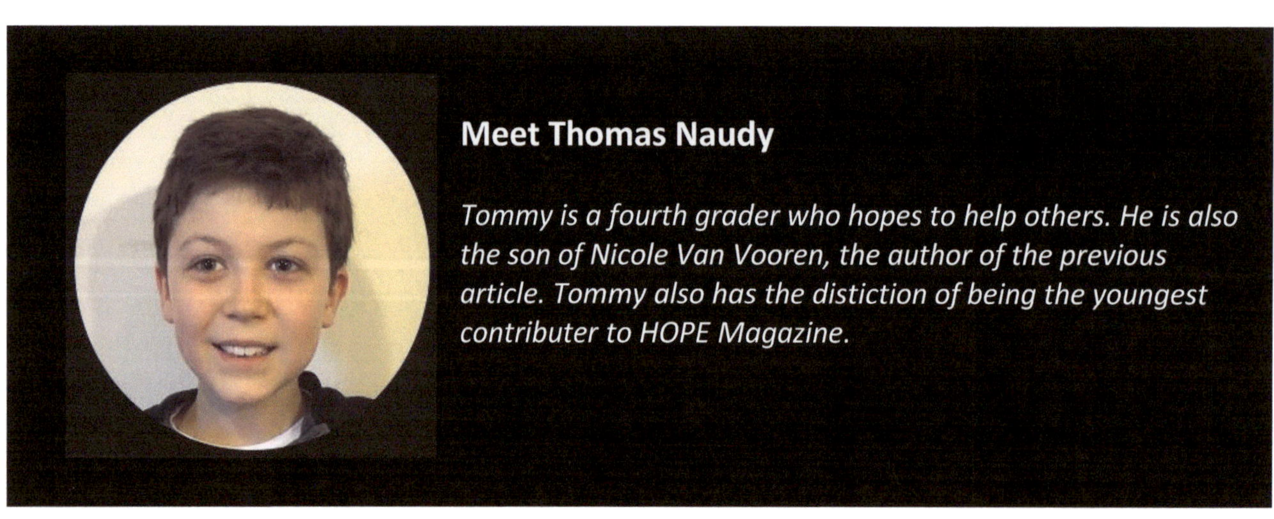

Meet Thomas Naudy

Tommy is a fourth grader who hopes to help others. He is also the son of Nicole Van Vooren, the author of the previous article. Tommy also has the distiction of being the youngest contributer to HOPE Magazine.

Join our Facebook Family

What do almost 30,000 people from 60 countries and five continents all have in common? They are all members of our vibrant Facebook family at **f**/TBIHopeandInspiration

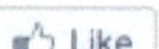

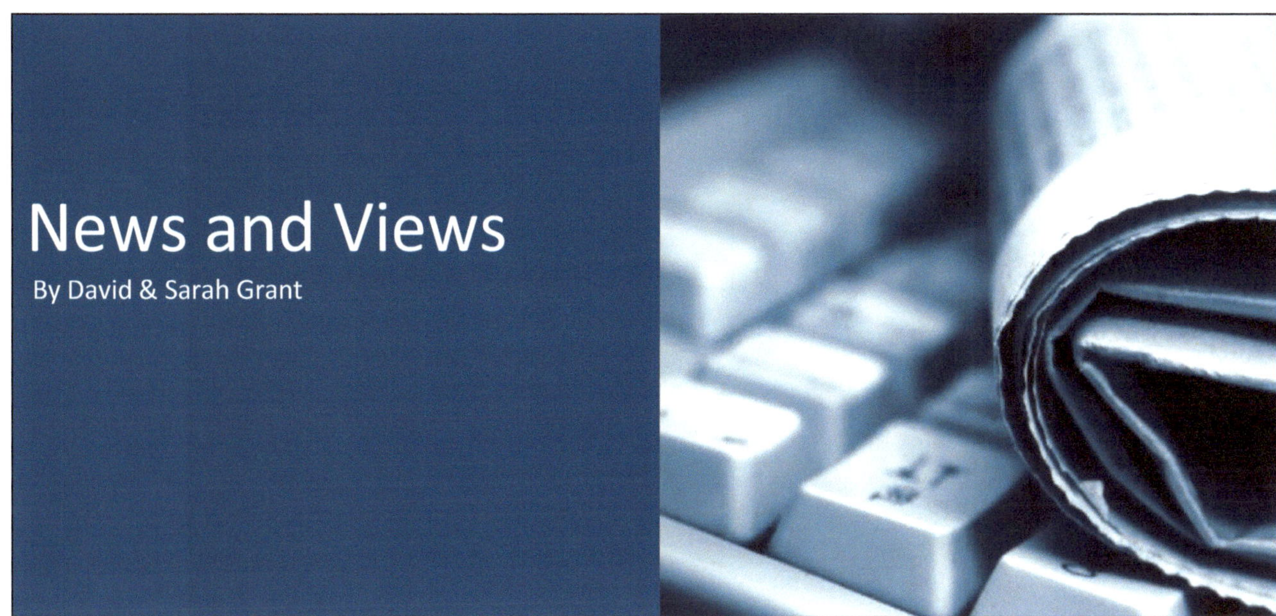

News and Views

By David & Sarah Grant

Over the years, we've known that our publication helps our readers to feel less alone, to know that their circumstances are not unique, and to feel a real and meaningful hope that life can be enjoyed and appreciated at a deep level after brain injury.

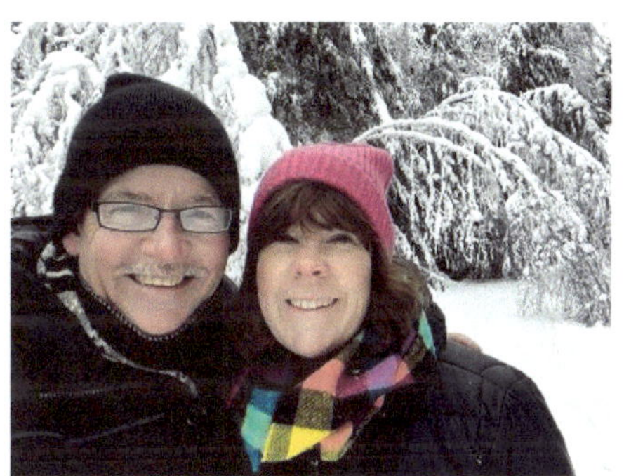

But we never gave much thought to how being part of HOPE Magazine would affect our contributors. Over the years, many of our contributors have reached out to us with thanks and in gratitude, knowing that their stories have helped to lift humanity higher, and in that lifting, they were lifted as well. Sharing their deep personal challenges has helped them to see that their experiences serve a greater good.

When I first read our last story, *Mommy's Brain Injury*, I must admit that I was a bit skeptical. How could one so young capture so eloquently the subtle nuances of life after brain injury. Included with his submission was a short video that his mom Nicole shot. His video started with, "Hi Dave…." and he went on to speak about his experiences. I was moved to tears.

Brain injury, like life itself these days, is not easy. So many are affected, but it often from the most innocent ones, those that we least expect, that comes the greatest of wisdom. To Tommy Naudy, I say, "Thank you. You are a courageous young man, one who would make any parent proud."

Together we can accomplish what none of us can do alone.

Be smart and stay safe.

~ David & Sarah